Access your Online Resources

Mindy and Mo's Crazy Carpet is accompanied by some downloadable material to help children practise the 'c' and 'k' sounds.

Go to https://resourcecentre.routledge.com/speechmark and click on the cover of this book.

Answer the question prompt using your copy of the book to gain access to the online content.

T0284181

Mindy and Mo's Crazy Carpet

Mindy and Mo love to play in a wood not far away. Join these two fun-loving adventurers as they loop the loop on a magic carpet over the desert and meet Carter who has a magic lamp. Can Mindy and Mo help Carter find the missing Carney Stone and free the genie Cabu before it's time to leave? What will the fallen tree be the next time they visit? And what will they see?

This Mindy and Mo story has been written to support children who are working on the 'c' and 'k' sounds. Support your child's practise of their target sound by sharing Mindy and Mo's adventure in the twinkling city of Cabok and encouraging them to join in with Mindy and Mo's 'carney, cackarney' call. Engaging characters and plot, supported by a rhythmic and rhyming structure, ensure this book not only supports speech development, but also entertains and inspires. Creatively and descriptively told, this story introduces new words and provides opportunities for developing literacy skills. Through positive characterisation, it also explores the themes of growth mindset, empathy, kindness and resilience, allowing children to make connections to their own lives and experiences.

A helpful section of suggested activities at the back of the book can be used to support further practise of the target speech sound. It also includes ideas for how this story can be used to help children to connect to nature through imagination. This humorous and triumphant story has been designed to support the individual child but is one which every child can enjoy!

Emily Kempster is an English teacher with 20 years' experience working in Gloucestershire secondary schools. Her passion for books inspired her to write from a young age, anything from short plays to ghost stories. More recently, in an attempt to entertain her young family and support her youngest daughter's difficulties with some speech sounds, she has focused on writing narrative poems. She hopes that the Mindy and Mo adventures will capture the imagination of young readers as well as support their speech sound development.

Lucy Cannon is a painter, illustrator and designer. Interested in all things creative from an early age, she studied Art and Graphic Design at college before heading into a successful management career in the voluntary sector. To follow her passion for art she set up Imagination by Lucy, which offers mural painting, illustration and creating custom home furnishings and apparel. Lucy is also involved in charity work, helping families who have children with heart conditions, but her most rewarding role to date is that of mum to two young children, one of whom had significant speech difficulties up to the age of 5. She now juggles time between bringing up her family, running her business, helping others and eating too much chocolate.

Rebecca Skinner is Head of Speech and Language Therapy and author at Thriving Language Community Interest Company. Co-founded by Rebecca and Becky Poulter Jewson, Thriving Language specialises in early years consultancy, offering training to early years settings and guest lecturing at universities on their undergraduate courses in Early Childhood Studies. Rebecca also works for the Gloucestershire Health and Care NHS Foundation Trust as a Specialist Speech and Language Therapist, specialising in early years and cleft palate.

Mindy and Mo's Crazy Carpet

Emily Kempster, Lucy Cannon and Rebecca Skinner

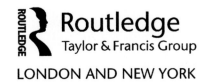

Routledge
Taylor & Francis Group

LONDON AND NEW YORK

Designed cover image: Lucy Cannon

First published 2025
by Routledge
4 Park Square, Milton Park, Abingdon, Oxon OX14 4RN

and by Routledge
605 Third Avenue, New York, NY 10158

Routledge is an imprint of the Taylor & Francis Group, an informa business

© 2025 Emily Kempster, Lucy Cannon and Rebecca Skinner

The right of Emily Kempster and Rebecca Skinner to be identified as authors and Lucy Cannon to be identified as illustrator of this work has been asserted in accordance with sections 77 and 78 of the Copyright, Designs and Patents Act 1988.

All rights reserved. No part of this book may be reprinted or reproduced or utilised in any form or by any electronic, mechanical, or other means, now known or hereafter invented, including photocopying and recording, or in any information storage or retrieval system, without permission in writing from the publishers.

Trademark notice: Product or corporate names may be trademarks or registered trademarks, and are used only for identification and explanation without intent to infringe.

British Library Cataloguing-in-Publication Data
A catalogue record for this book is available from the British Library

Library of Congress Cataloging-in-Publication Data
A catalog record has been requested for this book

ISBN: 978-1-032-85900-2 (pbk)
ISBN: 978-1-003-52039-9 (ebk)

DOI: 10.4324/9781003520399

This book can also be purchased as part of a set:
The Adventures of Mindy and Mo
ISBN: 978-1-032-43693-7 (pbk set)

Typeset in Futura Std
by Deanta Global Publishing Services, Chennai, India

Access the Support Material: https://resourcecentre.routledge.com/speechmark

Contents

Guidance for the Reader

We really hope you enjoy this Mindy and Mo adventure. There are seven others for you to read.

This series has been created by Rebecca Skinner, Specialist Speech and Language Therapist, Emily Kempster and Lucy Cannon in order to promote listening and awareness of specific speech sounds.

This book is loaded with the target sound 'c'/ 'k', giving the reader opportunities to model this sound naturally to children.

Each Mindy and Mo story includes a fun chorus containing 'nonsense words'. Not knowing these words or having a pre-existing way of saying them, makes it easier for children to practise blending their 'tricky sound' into a word structure. Children may like to join you in saying the chorus as they become familiar with the story.

Sharing this book with children who are having difficulty with the sound 'c'/ 'k' is a non-direct intervention, enabling you to support speech sound development in a fun way, without putting any pressure on the child.

These stories can be enjoyed by **all** children, enabling speech sound intervention to be fully inclusive.

Top tips

- Enjoy the story – children love to engage with stories and characters. This book can be enjoyed by all children.

- Talk naturally – you don't need to emphasise the target sound.

- Re-visit the story – you can raise the child's awareness of the target sound, for example 'carney, cackarney' – "that starts with a 'c'" (remember that we are talking about the sound 'c'/ 'k' and not the letter 'kuh', or 'kay').

- Draw the child's attention to your mouth when you are talking about the target sound – "look at my mouth when I say 'c'/ 'k', the back of my tongue is tapping against the back of my mouth".

- Extend the experience – support children to use the ideas in the story to develop their imagination and vocabulary. When you are outside you might find a fallen tree or a 'magic tree' – where would you and your children like to go on your adventure?

Meet the Characters

 Hi, I'm Mindy! I'm pleased you're coming on an adventure with me and my friend Mo. We love playing outside, especially at the fallen tree – it's our favourite place. How the tree came to fall down, we don't know, but we do know that in our imagination we can turn it into whatever we like. Come on! Let's see where it takes us.

 Hi, I'm Mo – that's short for Morris. I love playing outside with Mindy at the fallen tree, it's always lots of fun. Sometimes I struggle to hear everything clearly, but my hearing aid helps with that. Outside noises are different to inside ones, I like them. Being outside helps me to hear better, especially when Mindy talks to me. I'm pleased you're coming to see the magical tree with us. Come on, let's explore.

 Don't forget me! I'm Sid the snail and I go on every adventure. See if you can spot me along the way.

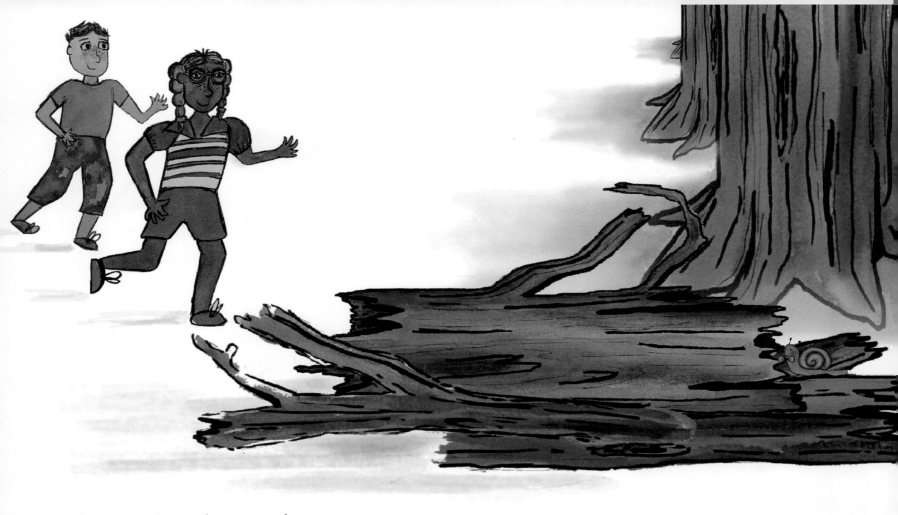

Mindy and Mo love to play
In a wood not far away.
They head straight for the fallen tree.
What will it be? What will they see?

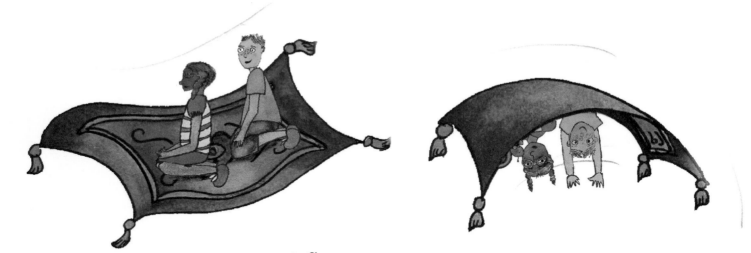

A flying carpet!

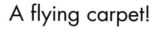

Quick, direct, the carpet zips,
Then like an acrobat it flips.
'Incredible!' Mindy calls out.
'Electrifying ride!' Mo shouts.

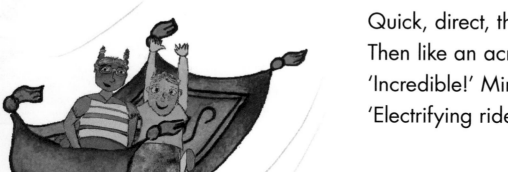

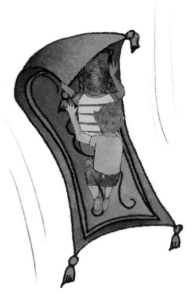

Across the desert, over rocks,
Past a scampering desert fox.
Above dark caves, secrets held tight,
And camels decked in colours bright.

'Mindy, look! Cabok's in view!'
The city twinkles, carpet zooms.
'There's Carter, Mo, what's in his hand?'
'I'm not too sure. It's time to land.'

'Carney, cackarney!
Come out Cabu!
Carney, cackarney!
Come out Cabu!'

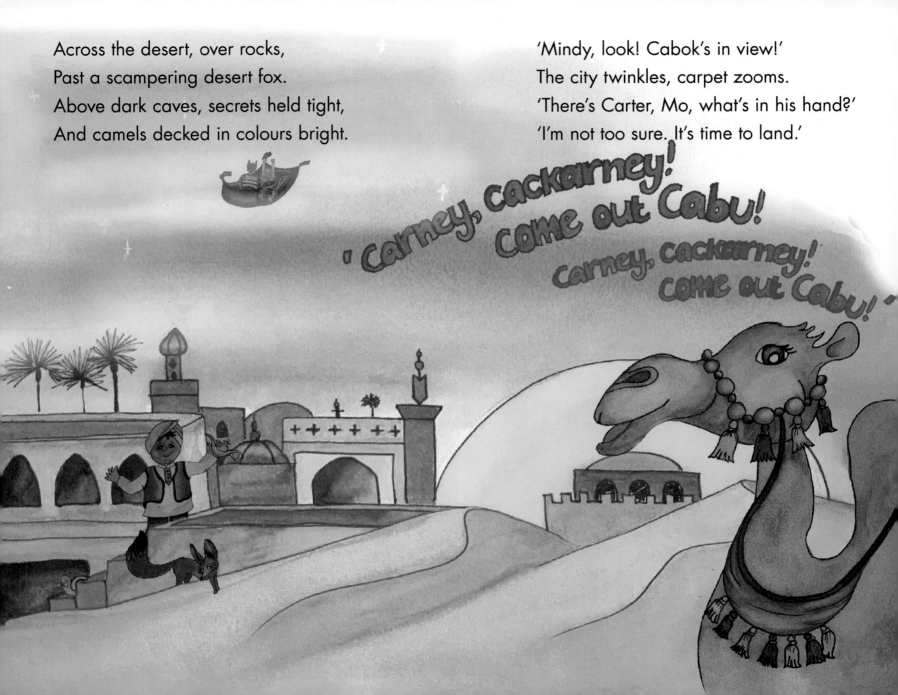

'Mindy, Mo, so pleased it's you.
Stuck in this lamp's the Great Cabu.
Someone took the Carney Stone;
This magic lamp can't work alone.'

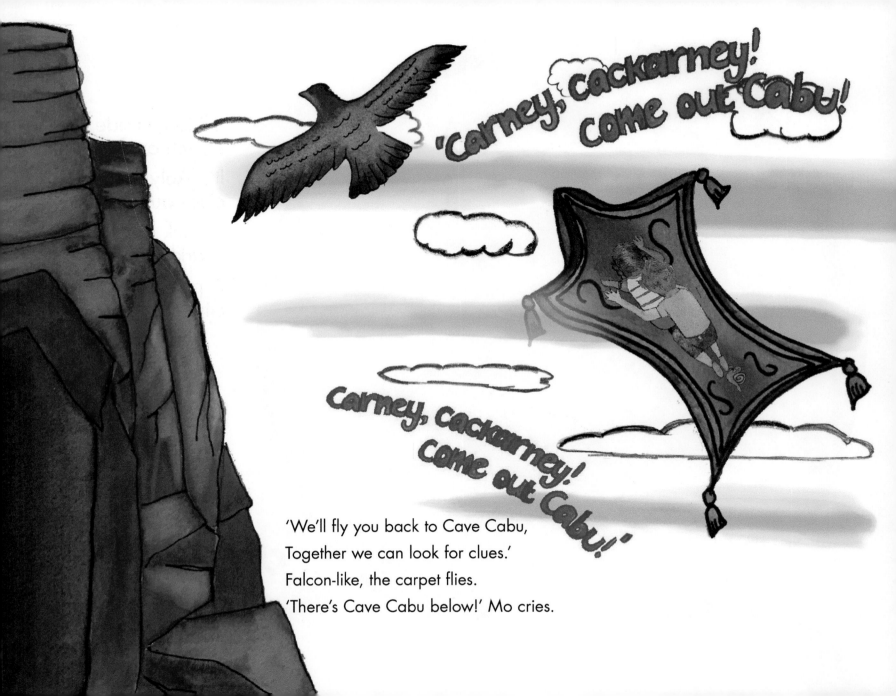

'We'll fly you back to Cave Cabu,
Together we can look for clues.'
Falcon-like, the carpet flies.
'There's Cave Cabu below!' Mo cries.

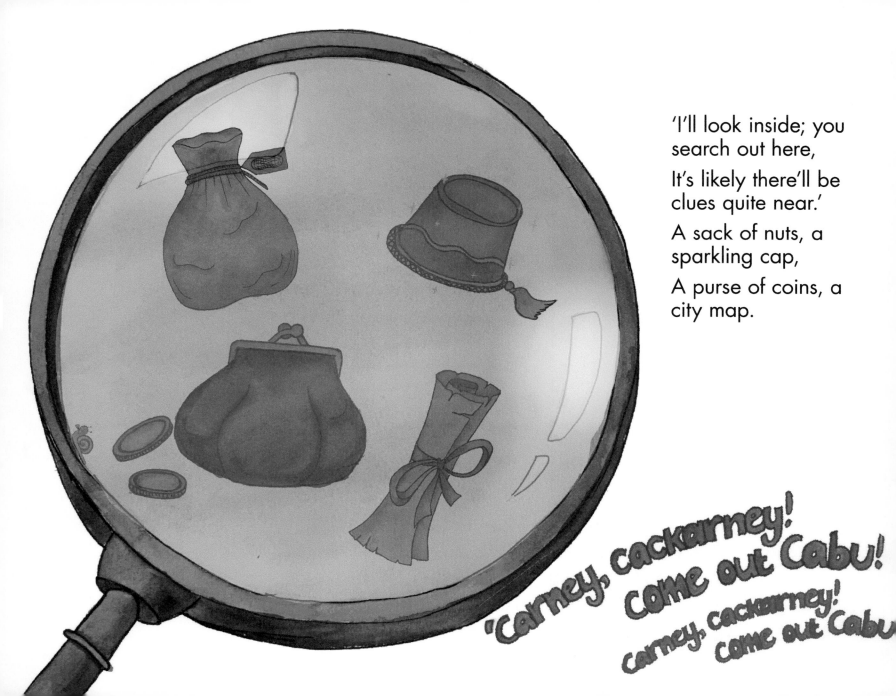

'I'll look inside; you search out here,

It's likely there'll be clues quite near.'

A sack of nuts, a sparkling cap,

A purse of coins, a city map.

'Carney, Cackarney! Come out Cabu!

Carney, cackarney! Come out Cabu!

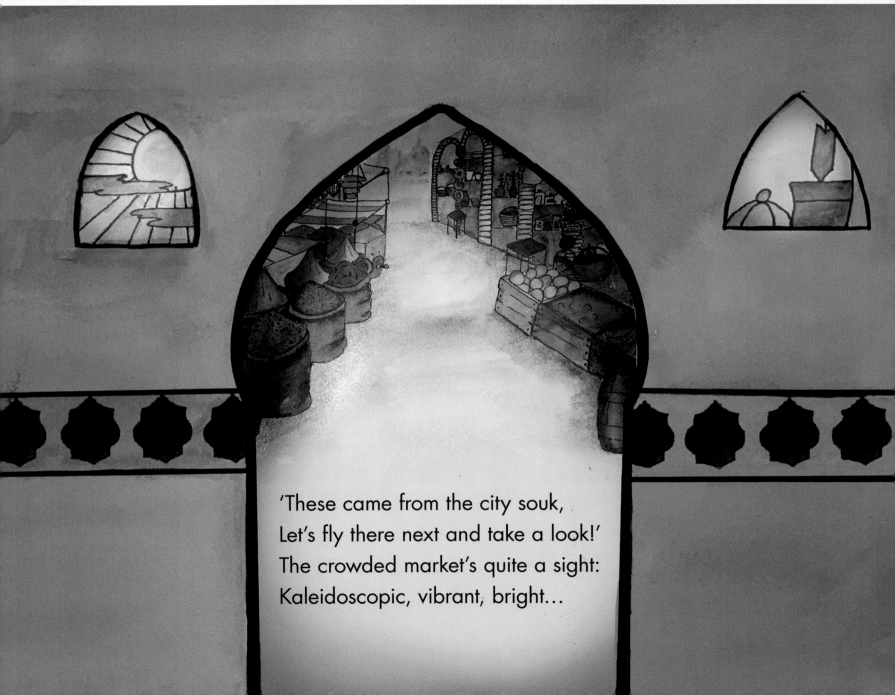

'These came from the city souk,
Let's fly there next and take a look!'
The crowded market's quite a sight:
Kaleidoscopic, vibrant, bright…

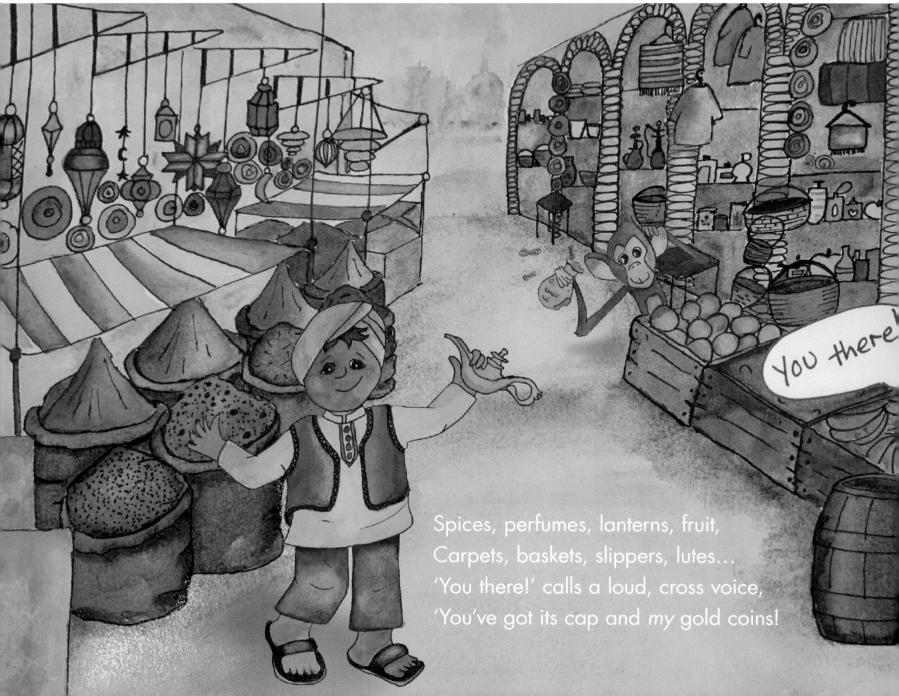

Spices, perfumes, lanterns, fruit,
Carpets, baskets, slippers, lutes…
'You there!' calls a loud, cross voice,
'You've got its cap and *my* gold coins!

'That monkey rascal's such a thief.
It's mischief quite beyond belief.
Objects shiny, sparkly, new,
It takes them all. What can I do?'

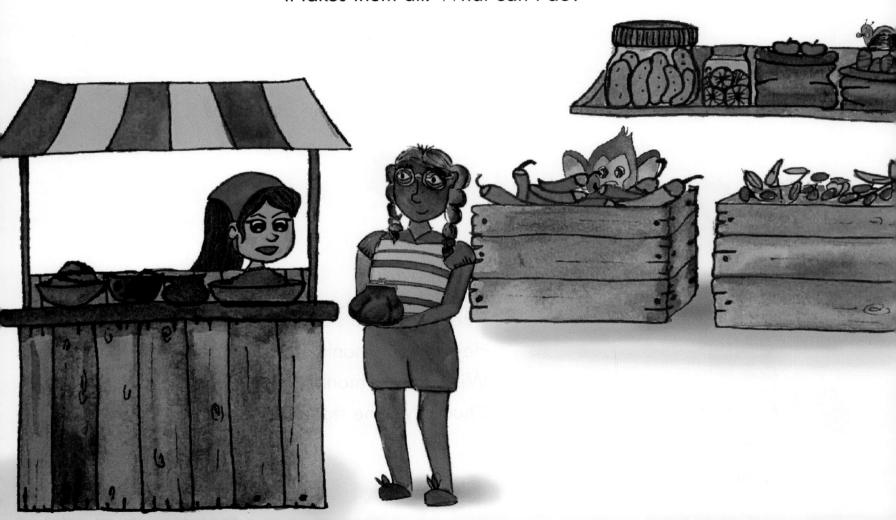

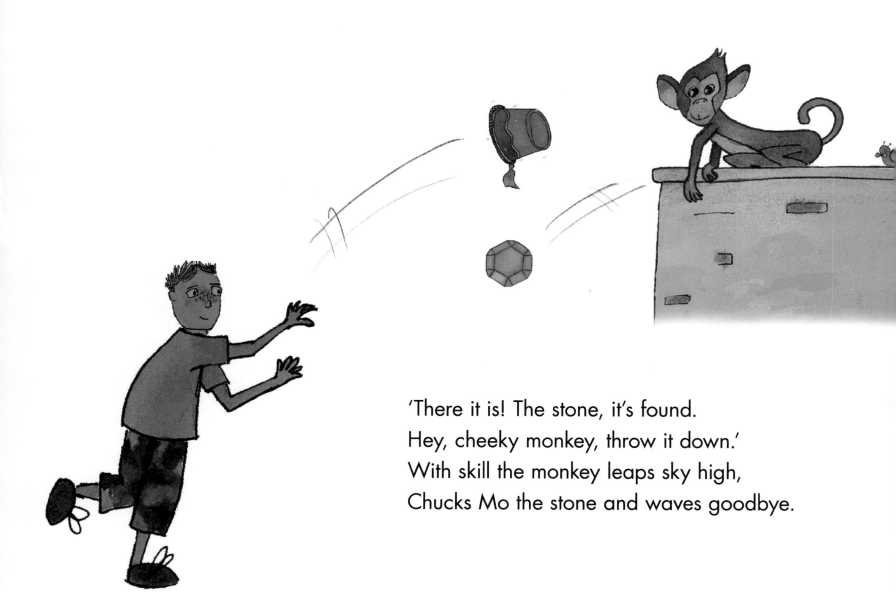

'There it is! The stone, it's found.
Hey, cheeky monkey, throw it down.'
With skill the monkey leaps sky high,
Chucks Mo the stone and waves goodbye.

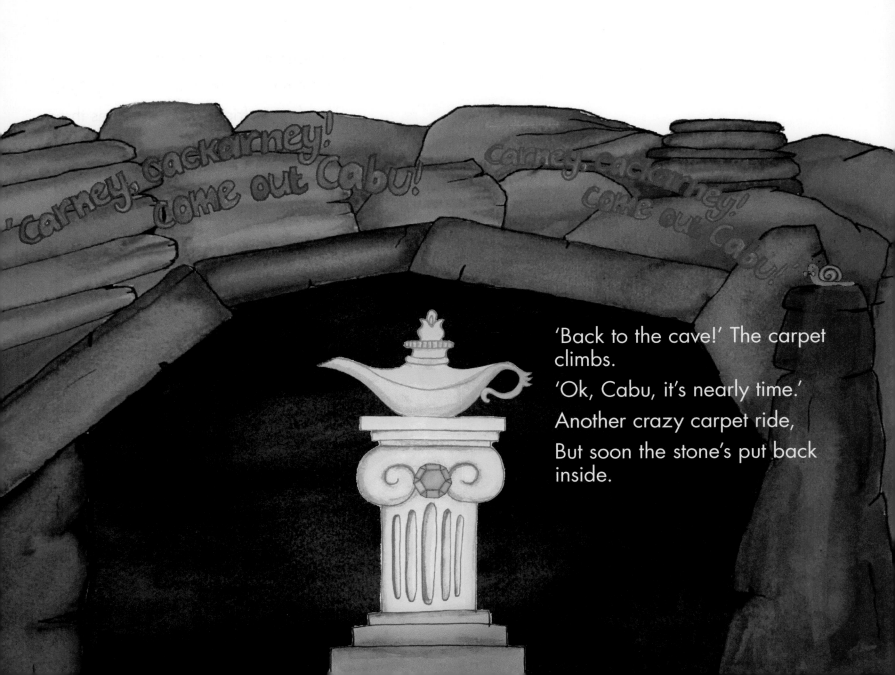

'Back to the cave!' The carpet climbs.

'Ok, Cabu, it's nearly time.'

Another crazy carpet ride,

But soon the stone's put back inside.

A colossal crash, gigantic cloud,
And then a voice, commanding, loud.
'Thank you, friends! Your wishes three
Are yours to make now that I'm free.'

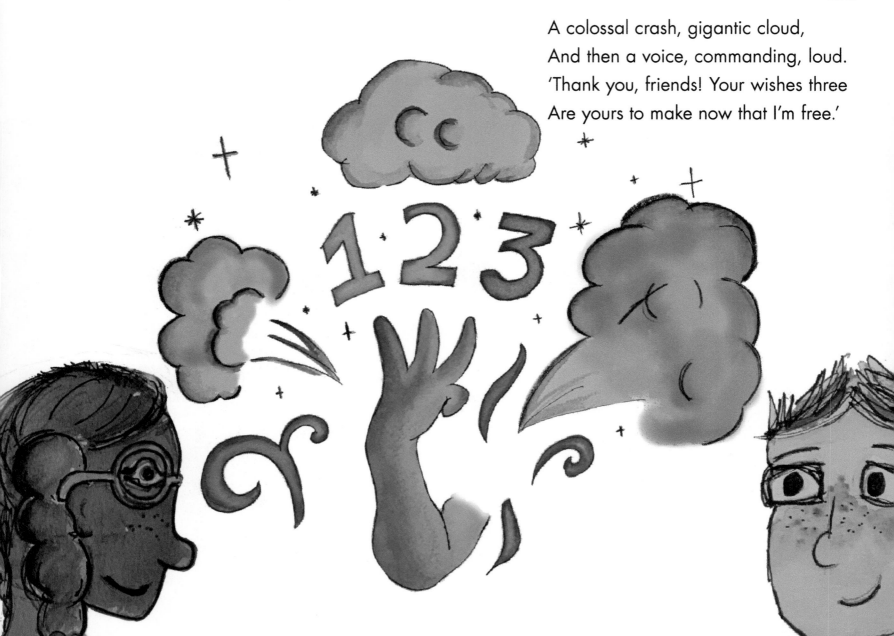

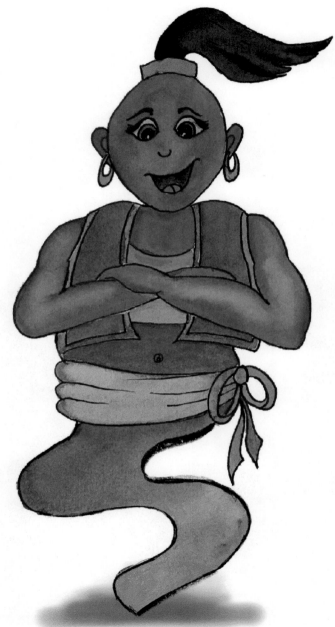

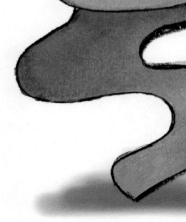

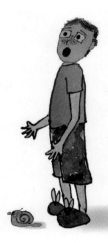

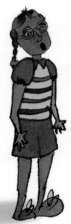

With curling smile and clever eyes,

A genie stands, three times their size.

First in lilac, then in pink,

A different colour with each blink.

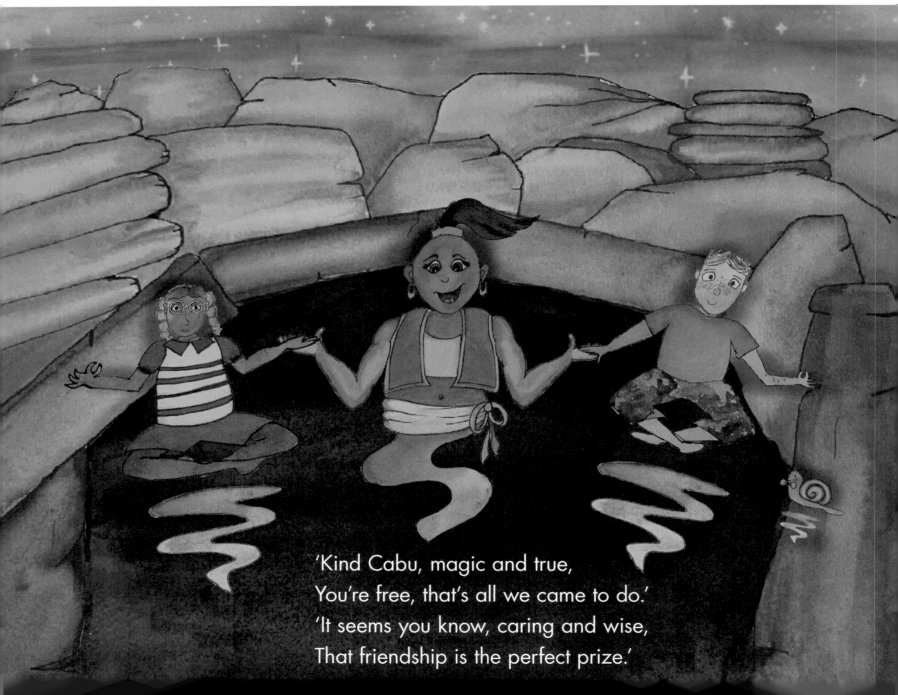

'Kind Cabu, magic and true,
You're free, that's all we came to do.'
'It seems you know, caring and wise,
That friendship is the perfect prize.'

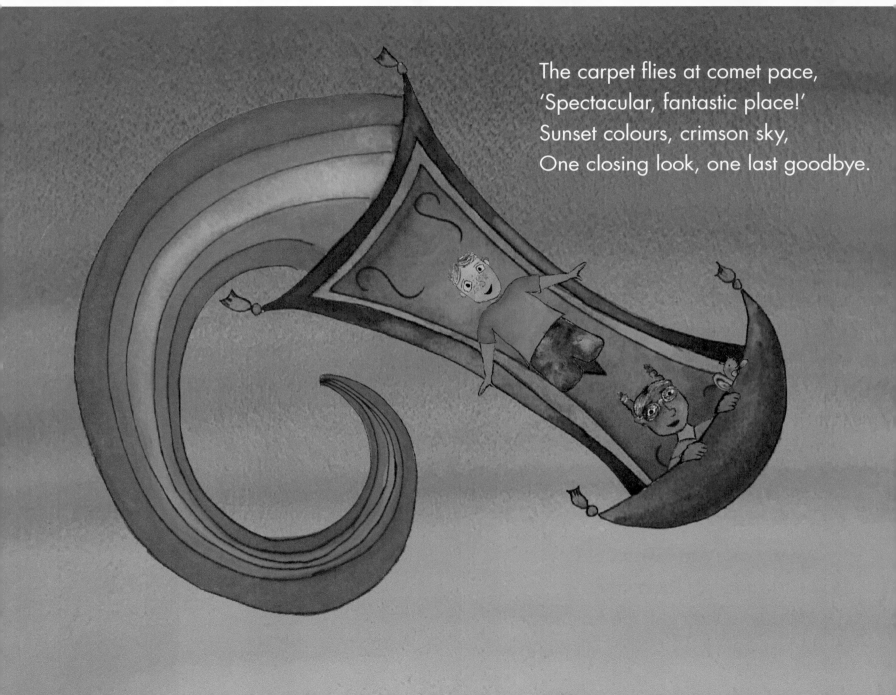

The carpet flies at comet pace,
'Spectacular, fantastic place!'
Sunset colours, crimson sky,
One closing look, one last goodbye.

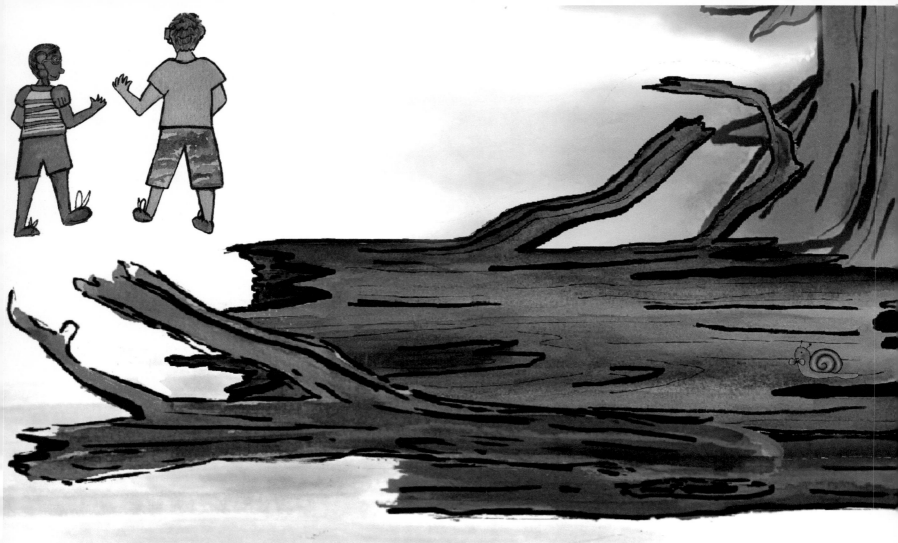

Mindy and Mo love to play
In a wood not far away.
Next time they visit the fallen tree,
What will it be? What will they see?

Further Activities: 'c'/ 'k'

We hope you enjoyed sharing in the adventures of Mindy and Mo. The aim of this book is to entertain children with a fun story which is loaded with the target sound 'c'/ 'k', providing them with opportunities to hear the sound and have a go.

Here are some further activities to support development of the sound 'c'/ 'k'.

How do we produce the sound 'c'/ 'k'?

The sound 'c'/ 'k' is a quiet sound. It is produced by lifting the back of the tongue up to the roof of the mouth, keeping the front of the tongue down. The back of the tongue taps against the roof of the mouth and this contact creates a pressure from which the sound can burst through the mouth.

Ways you can promote the target sound 'c'/ 'k'

- **Go on a sound hunt**
  Look around your environment for objects which start with a 'c'/ 'k' (car), have a 'c'/ 'k' in the middle (basket) or a 'c'/ 'k' at the end of the word (book). Remember we are talking about the sound and not the letter. As you find your objects, talk about them together to raise your child's awareness of the sound 'c'/ 'k' in the word.

- **Find the 'c'/ 'k'**
  Gather a pile of objects or pictures, some of which start with the sound 'c'/ 'k' and others starting with different sounds. Together find all the items which start with a 'c'/ 'k'. Select one item at a time, say the word and think aloud: does it start with a 'c'/ 'k'? If the child is struggling to say the sound 'c'/ 'k' accurately, say the word to them so they can hear the sound modelled.

- **Hide and seek**
  Collect pictures of objects that start with a 'c'/ 'k', have a 'c'/ 'k' in the middle or a 'c'/ 'k' at the end of the word. Take turns to hide the pictures in different places in your environment while the other person closes their eyes. Name the pictures as you find them. Remember you will need to model the words if the child is struggling to say the sound 'c'/ 'k'.

Important

These activities should be fun, so please remember not to put pressure on the child to say the sound. Enjoy the book and use the activities to model the target sound and support speech sound development.

More ways in which this book can be enjoyed and encourage your child to imagine, explore and learn

1. Head outside and find a tree. Use your imagination: What could the tree become? Where could it take you? What could you see and do there?

2. What does a tree need to grow? How does a tree change each season? How do trees feel when you touch them?

3. The genie Cabu tells Mindy and Mo that friendship is the perfect prize. What makes a good friend?

Word List

Words starting with 'c'/ 'k'	Words with 'c'/ 'k' in the middle	Words ending with 'c'/ 'k'
Car	Looking	Back
Cup	Basket	Sack
Key	Bucket	Pink
Can	Chicken	Blink
Cap	Acorn	Look
Coin	Monkey	Park